Neurogenesis Diet

A Beginner's 3-Week Step-by-Step Guide to Optimize Brain Health, with Curated Recipes and a Sample Meal Plan

mf

copyright © 2021 Larry Jamesonn

All rights reserved No part of this book may be reproduced, or stored in a retrieval system, or transmitted in any form or by any means, electronic, mechanical, photocopying, recording, or otherwise, without express written permission of the publisher.

Disclaimer

By reading this disclaimer, you are accepting the terms of the disclaimer in full. If you disagree with this disclaimer, please do not read the guide.

All of the content within this guide is provided for informational and educational purposes only, and should not be accepted as independent medical or other professional advice. The author is not a doctor, physician, nurse, mental health provider, or registered nutritionist/dietician. Therefore, using and reading this guide does not establish any form of a physician-patient relationship.

Always consult with a physician or another qualified health provider with any issues or questions you might have regarding any sort of medical condition. Do not ever disregard any qualified professional medical advice or delay seeking that advice because of anything you have read in this guide. The information in this guide is not intended to be any sort of medical advice and should not be used in lieu of any medical advice by a licensed and qualified medical professional.

The information in this guide has been compiled from a variety of known sources. However, the author cannot attest to or guarantee the accuracy of each source and thus should not be held liable for any errors or omissions.

You acknowledge that the publisher of this guide will not be held liable for any loss or damage of any kind incurred as a result of this guide or the reliance on any information provided within this guide. You acknowledge and agree that you assume all risk and responsibility for any action you undertake in response to the information in this guide.

Using this guide does not guarantee any particular result (e.g., weight loss or a cure). By reading this guide, you acknowledge that there are no guarantees to any specific outcome or results you can expect.

All product names, diet plans, or names used in this guide are for identification purposes only and are the property of their respective owners. The use of these names does not imply endorsement. All other trademarks cited herein are the property of their respective owners.

Where applicable, this guide is not intended to be a substitute for the original work of this diet plan and is, at most, a supplement to the original work for this diet plan and never a direct substitute. This guide is a personal expression of the facts of that diet plan.

Where applicable, persons shown in the cover images are stock photography models and the publisher has obtained the rights to use the images through license agreements with third-party stock image companies.

Table of Contents

Introduction   7
Understanding Neurogenesis   10
   Impact on Learning, Memory, and Mood   10
   Factors Influencing Neurogenesis   11
Defining the Neurogenesis Diet   13
   Principles of the Neurogenesis Diet   13
   Benefits of the Neurogenesis Diet   15
   Disadvantages of the Neurogenesis Diet   17
Your Ideal Neurogenesis Ingredients   19
   Blueberries   20
   Raspberry Blueberry Smoothie   21
   Blueberry Flax Smoothie   22
   Salmon   23
   Salmon Salad   24
   Braised Salmon with a Green Tea Mango Blast   25
   Hot, hot, hot Salmon   26
   Green Tea   27
   Matcha Green Tea Latte   28
   Curcumin   29
   Avocado, Cucumber, and Tomato Salad   30
   Cod Pea Curry   31
5-Step-by-Step Guide to Get Started with the Neurogenesis Diet   33
   Step 1: Educate Yourself   33
   Step 2: Plan Your Meals   34
   Step 3: Stock Your Kitchen   36
   Step 4: Prepare Healthy Recipes   38
   Step 5: Monitor and Adjust Your Diet   41
   Practical Tips for Shopping   44

Foods to Eat	47
Foods to Avoid	50
Foods and Habits to Avoid	**53**
Week 1 – Meal and Stomach Prep	**55**
Start with your gut	55
Week 2 – Going Full Swing	**59**
Taking a Holistic Approach	59
Add Aerobic Exercise	59
Caloric Restriction	60
Sleep	61
Week 3 – Sustainability and Discipline	**64**
Set realistic goals (beyond the 3-week plan)	64
Remove unhealthy foods from your house	65
Track your progress	66
More Meal Ideas	**68**
Salmon with Avocados and Brussels Sprouts	69
Salmon Soup	70
Tortilla Wraps	71
French Toast	72
Grilled Beef Burger	73
Pesto-Sauce Noodles	74
Waffles Topped with Peanut Butter and Blueberry Jam	75
Garden Greens Salad	77
Chicken Curry	78
Conclusion	**80**
FAQs	**83**
References and Helpful Links	**86**

Introduction

Neurogenesis, the process of forming new neurons in the brain, has captured the interest of scientists and health enthusiasts. For decades, it was believed that the brain's neuron count was fixed by early adulthood, but recent discoveries have debunked this myth. Neurogenesis continues throughout life and can be influenced by various factors, including diet. This guide delves into the science of neurogenesis and introduces a diet plan designed to support this crucial brain function.

Understanding neurogenesis starts with recognizing its importance. Neurons are the brain's building blocks, responsible for processing and transmitting information. The continuous formation of new neurons is essential for cognitive functions, emotional well-being, and overall brain health.

But what if there was a way to naturally stimulate this process? Research indicates that certain dietary choices can foster neurogenesis, offering a practical approach to brain health.

This guide explores the relationship between food and neurogenesis, offering insights into how specific nutrients and eating habits can boost brain health. It covers foods rich in neurogenic properties, from leafy greens and berries to omega-3-rich fish and nuts. Each section explains why these foods are beneficial and how they contribute to neuron growth and repair.

For those seeking to enhance their mental clarity, memory, or emotional resilience, the Neurogenesis Diet Guide offers a tailored approach to dietary wellness. Grounded in scientific research, it presents actionable advice that is easy to incorporate into daily life. By following the recommendations in this guide, individuals can take proactive steps toward improving brain health through mindful eating.

This is not about drastic changes or restrictive diets; instead, it emphasizes balanced, nutrient-dense foods that support the brain's natural processes. The guide also includes practical tips for meal planning, shopping lists, and simple recipes that make integrating neurogenic foods into your diet effortless. Whether one is a seasoned health enthusiast or just beginning their journey towards better brain health, this guide serves as a valuable resource.

In the Neurogenesis Diet 3-Week Plan, you'll discover:

- How to get into the Neurogenesis Diet

- The phenomenal wonders your body can achieve by getting into this
- How to make a lifestyle of this diet
- Holistic routine tweaks that get you the best results
- Simple meals or snacks you can make for the diet
- What good fat-rich foods can you make at home
- Tips for sustaining a new diet
- How you can stay healthy for decades to come

Ready to embark on a journey towards optimal brain health? The Neurogenesis Diet Guide is designed to provide everything needed to understand and apply the principles of neurogenesis in daily life. Join countless others who have discovered the benefits of supporting their brain through thoughtful dietary choices. Begin exploring this guide today and take the first step towards nourishing your brain for a healthier, more vibrant future.

Understanding Neurogenesis

Neurogenesis is the process by which new neurons are formed in the brain. This phenomenon primarily occurs in the hippocampus, a region associated with learning, memory, and emotion. The significance of neurogenesis lies in its potential to enhance cognitive functions and overall brain health. By generating new neurons, the brain can improve its capacity for learning, strengthen memory retention, and regulate mood more effectively.

Impact on Learning, Memory, and Mood

Neurogenesis plays a pivotal role in enhancing various cognitive functions and emotional states. Here's how it specifically impacts learning, memory, and mood:

- *Learning*: Neurogenesis supports the brain's ability to absorb and retain new information. New neurons contribute to the creation of neural circuits that are essential for processing and storing knowledge.
- *Memory*: The formation of new neurons aids in the consolidation of short-term memories into long-term ones. This process ensures that experiences and

learned information are more permanently integrated into our cognitive framework.
- *Mood*: Neurogenesis has been linked to emotional regulation and mental well-being. Increased neurogenesis can help alleviate symptoms of depression and anxiety by promoting a balanced production of neurotransmitters that affect mood.

Neurogenesis, therefore, is a fundamental process that not only bolsters our cognitive abilities but also plays a crucial role in maintaining emotional balance and mental health.

Factors Influencing Neurogenesis

Several lifestyle factors can significantly influence the rate and effectiveness of neurogenesis, including:

- *Exercise*: Physical activity, especially aerobic exercises like running or swimming, has been shown to stimulate the production of new neurons. Exercise increases blood flow to the brain, providing the necessary oxygen and nutrients for neurogenesis.
- *Sleep*: Quality sleep is essential for neurogenesis. During sleep, the brain undergoes repair and maintenance processes that facilitate the growth of new neurons. Adequate rest ensures optimal brain function and enhances cognitive performance.
- *Diet*: Nutrition plays a crucial role in supporting neurogenesis. Consuming a diet rich in specific

nutrients, such as omega-3 fatty acids, antioxidants, flavonoids, and B vitamins, can promote the growth of new neurons and protect existing brain cells from damage.

Understanding these factors and their impact on neurogenesis provides a foundation for adopting habits that can enhance brain health and cognitive function.

Defining the Neurogenesis Diet

From the '60s through the '80s, the scientific community believed that once a person reached adulthood, neuron and brain tissue growth halted significantly (Mandal, 2019). However, recent studies confirm that neurogenesis continues throughout life.

Most doctors and fitness experts today recommend physical exercise and a well-balanced diet for a healthy life. There are various physical activities and diets, each offering perks depending on your goals. However, the benefits of a neurogenesis diet stand out, particularly for the brain, the most important organ in the human body. In the next section, we will discuss the principles, benefits, and potential drawbacks of the neurogenesis diet.

Principles of the Neurogenesis Diet

To effectively support neurogenesis, the diet should focus on several key principles:

1. ***Rich in Omega-3 Fatty Acids***: Include foods high in omega-3 fatty acids like fatty fish (salmon, mackerel,

sardines), flaxseeds, chia seeds, and walnuts. These are essential for neuron membrane health and function.

2. *Abundant in Antioxidants*: Consume a variety of fruits and vegetables rich in antioxidants, such as berries (blueberries, strawberries, blackberries), leafy greens (spinach, kale), and cruciferous vegetables (broccoli, Brussels sprouts). Antioxidants protect neurons from oxidative stress and inflammation.

3. *High in Flavonoids*: Incorporate foods like dark chocolate, citrus fruits, apples, and green tea. Flavonoids promote the growth of new neurons and improve cognitive functions.

4. *B Vitamin-Rich Foods*: Ensure your diet includes foods high in B vitamins (B6, B12, folate) such as eggs, legumes, leafy greens, and fortified cereals. B vitamins are crucial for brain metabolism and neurogenesis.

5. *Adequate Magnesium and Zinc*: Include sources of magnesium (nuts, seeds, whole grains) and zinc (pumpkin seeds, chickpeas, shellfish). These minerals are vital for brain health and neuron development.

6. *Balanced Protein Intake*: Opt for lean proteins like chicken, turkey, beans, and lentils. Proteins provide amino acids necessary for neurotransmitter production and overall brain function.

7. *Minimize Processed Foods and Sugars*: Avoid excessive consumption of processed foods, sugars, and

trans fats, which can impair cognitive function and hinder neurogenesis.
8. *Hydrate Well*: Maintain proper hydration with water and herbal teas. Dehydration can negatively affect cognitive performance and overall brain health.
9. *Incorporate Healthy Fats*: Use healthy fats such as olive oil, avocados, and nuts to support brain cell integrity and function.

By adhering to these principles, the neurogenesis diet aims to enhance brain health, improve cognitive functions, and promote emotional well-being.

Benefits of the Neurogenesis Diet

The potential benefits of following the neurogenesis diet go beyond just improving brain health. Some of the additional benefits include:

1. *Enhanced Cognitive Function*: Boosts the brain's ability to learn, process information, and solve problems, leading to improved overall intellectual performance.
2. *Better Memory Retention*: Aids in the conversion of short-term memories into long-term storage, ensuring that experiences and information are more effectively retained and recalled.
3. *Mood Regulation*: Supports the balance of neurotransmitters, which can help reduce symptoms of

depression and anxiety, leading to more stable and positive emotional health.

4. ***Reduced Oxidative Stress***: Antioxidant-rich foods in the diet protect brain cells from damage caused by free radicals, reducing inflammation and slowing the aging process of the brain.
5. ***Improved Brain Plasticity***: Enhances the brain's ability to reorganize and form new neural connections, which is vital for learning, memory, and recovery from brain injuries.
6. ***Increased Neuron Formation***: Promotes the growth of new neurons, particularly in the hippocampus, enhancing overall brain health and cognitive function.
7. ***Protection Against Neurodegenerative Diseases***: Provides neuroprotective nutrients that may lower the risk of diseases such as Alzheimer's and Parkinson's, helping to maintain long-term brain health.
8. ***Better Emotional Stability***: Contributes to a well-balanced mental state by supporting neurogenesis linked to mood regulation, resulting in improved emotional resilience and stability.
9. ***Optimal Brain Metabolism***: Ensures efficient energy use and nutrient supply to brain cells, promoting peak brain function and preventing cognitive decline.
10. ***Enhanced Focus and Concentration***: Improves attention span and mental clarity, helping individuals to stay focused and productive in their daily tasks.

By incorporating brain-healthy foods into one's diet, individuals can not only improve their physical health but also support their cognitive function and emotional well-being. It is important to remember that a balanced and varied diet, along with regular exercise and good sleep habits, are essential for maintaining overall brain health.

Disadvantages of the Neurogenesis Diet

While the Neurogenesis Diet offers numerous benefits for brain health and cognitive function, it also has some disadvantages that should be considered:

1. ***Restrictive Dietary Choices***: Followers may find it challenging to adhere strictly to the recommended foods, limiting their variety and potentially making meal planning more complex.
2. ***Higher Cost***: The diet often includes high-quality, nutrient-dense foods like fatty fish, organic vegetables, and nuts, which can be more expensive than processed or conventional alternatives.
3. ***Time-Consuming Preparation***: Preparing meals with fresh, whole ingredients requires more time and effort compared to convenience foods, which might be difficult for individuals with busy schedules.
4. ***Potential Nutrient Imbalance***: Without careful planning, there is a risk of missing out on certain

essential nutrients, especially if the diet excludes certain food groups entirely.
5. ***Initial Adjustment Period***: Individuals may experience a period of adjustment where they feel low energy or other minor discomforts as their bodies adapt to the new diet.

Despite these disadvantages, the benefits of the Neurogenesis Diet, such as enhanced cognitive function, better memory retention, mood regulation, and protection against neurodegenerative diseases, significantly outweigh the drawbacks.

Your Ideal Neurogenesis Ingredients

As mentioned earlier, the best foods you can eat for the Neurogenesis diet are rich in omega-3 fatty acids, polyphenols, and resveratrol. Foods with vitamins B6 & B12 are excellent as well (Cortright, 2015). But one of the great things about adopting this diet is that it isn't heavily restrictive and does not cut out entire food groups.

There is plenty of room for creativity when preparing meals and snacks you can eat to induce neurogenesis. You can still make something in the kitchen that can up your mood and stimulate this process. After all, a positive one is helpful for neurogenesis (Stangl & Thuret, 2009).

However, if you're looking for the four best foods you can eat for this diet, these would be blueberries, fish that's rich in omega-3 fatty acids, green tea, and turmeric (Poulose et al., 2017).

Let's take a look at each one of these.

Blueberries

These blue or purple fruits are rich in polyphenols. Polyphenols are antioxidants that reduce oxidative stress (Tapeiro et al., 2002). Since there is a high oxygen demand for our brain functions, it is most susceptible to the effects of oxidative stress, the prime cause of neurodegenerative diseases such as Alzheimer's disease and Parkinson's disease (Kim et al., 2015).

By simply adding these humble, round fruits to your meals, you're already preventing neuron cell deterioration and giving way to the creation of new ones.

You also get the benefit of its flexibility as an ingredient for many dishes. Whether you're making a dessert, a salad, or a savory spread with blueberry jam, you can be creative with your diet options.

Here are just some fun, creative blueberry recipes you can try:

Raspberry Blueberry Smoothie

Ingredients:

- 1 cup frozen raspberries
- ½ cup frozen blueberries
- 1 banana
- ½ cup almond milk
- ¼ cup Greek yogurt
- 1 tablespoon honey (optional)

Instructions:

1. In a blender, combine all ingredients and blend until smooth.
2. If the consistency is too thick, add more almond milk or water to achieve your desired thickness.
3. Pour into a glass and enjoy!

Blueberry Flax Smoothie

Ingredients:

- 1 cup frozen blueberries
- 1 banana
- ½ cup almond milk
- ¼ cup Greek yogurt
- 1 tablespoon flax seeds

Instructions:

1. In a blender, combine all ingredients and blend until smooth.
2. Pour into a glass and sprinkle some additional flax seeds on top for added texture.
3. Serve and enjoy!

Salmon

Next on the list is this healthy fish which is commonly colored orange or red on the inside. It boasts being a rich source of omega-3 fatty acids. Consuming salmon benefits our brains by supplying the healthy fats needed for the continual development of its structure. Our brains consist of up to 60% fat after all (Syn, 2017). The omega-3 provided by salmon is one of the best qualities you can get and is key to increasing neurogenesis.

The following are delicious salmon-based dishes you can prepare at home:

Salmon Salad

Ingredients:

- 1 fresh salmon fillet
- Salad greens (spinach, arugula, kale)
- Cherry tomatoes
- Cucumber slices
- Avocado chunks

For dressing:

- olive oil
- lemon juice
- honey
- Dijon mustard

Instructions:

1. Grill or pan-fry the salmon until cooked to your liking.
2. Arrange salad greens in a bowl or on a plate.
3. Add cherry tomatoes, cucumber slices, and avocado chunks on top of the salad greens.
4. Place the cooked salmon fillet on top of the salad.
5. Drizzle with dressing and serve.

For dressing:

Mix olive oil, lemon juice, honey, and Dijon mustard.

Braised Salmon with a Green Tea Mango Blast

Ingredients:

- 1 fresh salmon fillet
- 1 tablespoon of green tea leaves or powder
- Salt and pepper to taste
- Olive oil for grilling

Instructions:

1. Rub the green tea leaves or powder all over the salmon fillet.
2. Season with salt and pepper.
3. Heat olive oil in a pan and grill the salmon until cooked through.
4. Serve with a side of mango salsa made by mixing diced mango, red onion, cilantro, lime juice, and chili flakes.

Hot, hot, hot Salmon

Ingredients:

- 1 fresh salmon fillet
- 2 tablespoons of honey
- 1 tablespoon of chili paste
- Salt and pepper to taste

Instructions:

1. Preheat your oven to 400°F.
2. Mix the honey, chili paste, salt, and pepper in a small bowl.
3. Place the salmon fillet on a baking sheet lined with foil.
4. Spread the honey-chili mixture evenly over the salmon fillet.
5. Bake for about 12 minutes or until the salmon flakes easily with a fork.

Green Tea

This soothing cup of tea comes from Camellia sinensis leaves and is also a great source of polyphenols, specifically Epigallocatechin-3-gallate (EGCG). ECCG is known to increase BDNF (brain-derived neurotrophic factor). It's also a key component of neurogenesis (Ding et al., 2017). It is also capable of improving learning and brain performance.

Sipping on this wondrous tea is an excellent option for whenever you're winding down after a long day of work.

To add a different twist to your usual tea brew, you can try the recipe below:

Matcha Green Tea Latte

Ingredients:

- 1 teaspoon of matcha green tea powder
- 1 cup of unsweetened almond milk
- Honey or agave syrup to taste

Instructions:

1. In a small saucepan, heat the almond milk until warm.
2. Add the matcha powder and whisk until smooth.
3. Optional: for a frothy texture, use a handheld frother or blender to blend the mixture.
4. Sweeten with honey or agave syrup to taste.
5. Serve hot and enjoy!

Curcumin

Curcumin is the main component found in turmeric. Turmeric alone is already jam-packed with known benefits to the human body. Curcumin benefits the brain by inducing powerful neurogenic effects alongside its anti-inflammatory and antioxidant properties. In aging populations, curcumin is a great way to prevent cognitive decline (Sarker & Franks, 2018).

It also goes into many dishes as a spice or as tea. You can try out curcumin in these simple dishes:

Avocado, Cucumber, and Tomato Salad

Ingredients:

- 1 avocado, diced
- 1 cucumber, peeled and sliced
- 1 cup cherry tomatoes, halved
- 2 tablespoons of olive oil
- Juice of half a lemon
- Salt and pepper to taste

Instructions:

1. In a large bowl, mix together the avocado, cucumber, and cherry tomatoes.
2. Drizzle olive oil and lemon juice over the salad.
3. Season with salt and pepper.
4. Toss until well combined.
5. Serve as a side dish or add protein for a complete meal.

Cod Pea Curry

Ingredients:

- 4 cod fillets, cut into chunks
- 1 cup frozen peas
- 1 onion, diced
- 2 cloves of garlic, minced
- 1 tablespoon olive oil
- 1 can of coconut milk
- 2 tablespoons of curry powder
- Salt and pepper to taste

Instructions:

1. In a large pan, heat olive oil over medium-high heat.
2. Add onions and cook until softened.
3. Add in the minced garlic and cook for an additional minute.
4. Stir in the curry powder and cook for 1-2 minutes.
5. Pour in the can of coconut milk and stir until well combined.
6. Add in the chunks of cod and frozen peas.
7. Let simmer for 10-15 minutes, or until fish is fully cooked and peas are tender.
8. Season with salt and pepper to taste.
9. Serve over rice or quinoa for a complete meal.

Those are just four of the best foods for the Neurogenesis diet. But you can also play around with these other options to add variety to your meal plan:

- Wild-caught Fish
- Grass-fed Beef
- Grass-fed dairy (milk)
- Cheese
- Pastured chicken & eggs
- Butter
- Nuts
- Mulberries
- Red Sage (Salvia)
- Goji Berries
- Pork Liver
- Clams

5-Step-by-Step Guide to Get Started with the Neurogenesis Diet

When it comes to incorporating the Neurogenesis diet into your lifestyle, it can be overwhelming at first. To help you get started, here is a simple 5-step guide that you can follow:

Step 1: Educate Yourself

Begin by diving deep into the principles and benefits of the Neurogenesis Diet. This diet focuses on foods that promote the growth and repair of neurons, enhancing overall brain health. First, understand the key nutrients essential for neurogenesis. These include omega-3 fatty acids, found in fatty fish like salmon and mackerel, crucial for maintaining brain cell structure and function.

Antioxidants protect brain cells from free radical damage. Foods rich in antioxidants include berries, dark chocolate, and green tea. Additionally, flavonoids, present in fruits, vegetables, and certain beverages like tea and red wine, support neurogenesis by enhancing blood flow to the brain and reducing inflammation.

To educate yourself, read scientific articles, books, and credible online resources about the Neurogenesis Diet. Understanding how these nutrients affect brain health will help you make informed dietary choices. Consult a nutritionist or dietitian for professional insights and personalized advice.

Knowledge is your foundation for success. As you learn more, take notes and create a reference guide for planning meals and grocery shopping. This preparation will help you transition smoothly into the Neurogenesis Diet and maximize its benefits for your cognitive and emotional well-being.

Step 2: Plan Your Meals

Creating a weekly meal plan is a crucial step in successfully adopting the Neurogenesis Diet. Start by identifying and integrating neurogenesis-friendly foods into your daily meals. These foods are rich in essential nutrients that support brain health, such as omega-3 fatty acids, antioxidants, and flavonoids.

Begin with fatty fish like salmon, mackerel, and sardines, which are excellent sources of omega-3 fatty acids. These can be included in your lunches and dinners, perhaps grilled, baked, or added to salads. Next, incorporate a variety of leafy greens such as spinach, kale, and Swiss chard. These vegetables are high in antioxidants and vitamins that protect brain cells from oxidative stress and inflammation. You can use them in salads, smoothies, or sautéed as side dishes.

Add berries like blueberries, strawberries, and blackberries to your breakfasts or snacks. Berries are packed with antioxidants and flavonoids known to enhance cognitive function and memory. They can be eaten fresh, added to yogurt, or blended into smoothies.

Nuts and seeds are another staple; walnuts, almonds, chia seeds, and flaxseeds provide not only omega-3s but also other essential fats and proteins that support brain health. These can be sprinkled on salads, mixed into oatmeal, or simply eaten as a snack.

To streamline your meal planning, draft a weekly meal plan that outlines each meal and snack. This helps ensure you're consistently incorporating these brain-boosting foods. For instance, plan for oatmeal topped with berries and nuts for breakfast, a leafy green salad with grilled salmon for lunch, and a dinner of quinoa paired with steamed veggies and a portion of mackerel.

Next, compile a detailed shopping list based on your meal plan. This list will include all the ingredients you need for the week, ensuring you have everything on hand and avoiding last-minute grocery trips. Group similar items together (e.g., fruits, vegetables, proteins) to make your shopping experience more efficient.

Additionally, consider prepping some ingredients in advance to save time during the week. Wash and chop vegetables, portion out nuts and seeds, and even pre-cook certain items like grains or proteins. This preparation can make following the diet more convenient and sustainable.

By organizing your meals and shopping systematically, you'll find it easier to stick to the Neurogenesis Diet, ultimately helping you reap its cognitive and emotional benefits.

Step 3: Stock Your Kitchen

To successfully follow the Neurogenesis Diet, it's essential to stock your kitchen with the right foods and ingredients. This preparation ensures that you have everything you need at your fingertips, making it easier to adhere to the diet and enjoy its numerous benefits for brain health.

1. *Fresh fruits*: Prioritize berries like blueberries, strawberries, and raspberries for their antioxidants and flavonoids that boost brain function. Other fruits like oranges, apples, and bananas provide essential vitamins and nutrients. Keep a variety to make your diet diverse and enjoyable.
2. *Vegetables*: Include leafy greens like spinach, kale, and Swiss chard, which are packed with vitamins and antioxidants crucial for brain health. Add cruciferous vegetables like broccoli and Brussels sprouts for their anti-inflammatory properties. Keep a mix of fresh,

frozen, and even canned options (with no added salt or sugar) to always have vegetables on hand.
3. ***Whole grains***: Make these the base of your meals. Stock up on quinoa, brown rice, oats, barley, and whole wheat products. These grains offer fiber, vitamins, and slow-releasing carbs that sustain energy and support brain health. Ensure variety to keep meals interesting and balanced.
4. ***Lean proteins***: Opt for high-quality sources such as fatty fish (salmon, mackerel, sardines), chicken, turkey, and plant-based options like legumes and tofu. These proteins provide essential amino acids and omega-3 fatty acids for neuron health. A variety of protein sources allows for diverse and satisfying meals.
5. ***Healthy fats***: Stock up on nuts and seeds such as walnuts, almonds, chia seeds, and flaxseeds. These are great for snacks or adding to salads, cereals, and smoothies. Also, have extra virgin olive oil and avocado oil for cooking and salads. These oils are rich in monounsaturated fats, which support brain health and reduce inflammation.
6. ***High-quality nutrient-dense foods***: Prioritize organic and sustainably sourced products when shopping to maximize nutritional value and minimize exposure to pesticides. Choosing high-quality ingredients improves brain health and overall well-being.

Don't forget to stock up on kitchen staples that make meal preparation convenient. These might include herbs and spices like turmeric, ginger, rosemary, and thyme, which have additional brain-boosting properties. Also, consider having healthy snacks like hummus, Greek yogurt, and dark chocolate (in moderation) to satisfy cravings while staying within the dietary guidelines.

By thoroughly stocking your kitchen with these essentials, you'll create an environment that supports your commitment to the Neurogenesis Diet, making it easier to prepare healthy, delicious meals that enhance your cognitive function and emotional well-being.

Step 4: Prepare Healthy Recipes

Creating delicious and nutritious meals is a key component of the Neurogenesis Diet. This step involves experimenting with new recipes that align with the principles of brain health. Here's how you can get started:

1. **Experiment with New Recipes**
   - *Diverse Ingredients*: Embrace a wide range of brain-boosting ingredients like fatty fish, leafy greens, nuts, seeds, berries, and whole grains. These foods are rich in omega-3 fatty acids, antioxidants, vitamins, and minerals that support cognitive function.

- *Culinary Exploration*: Don't be afraid to try new flavors and cuisines. Exploring different cooking techniques and ingredient combinations can make healthy eating more enjoyable and sustainable.

2. **Cooking Techniques**
   - *Simple Preparations*: Start with simple recipes that don't require extensive cooking skills. Over time, you can gradually tackle more complex dishes as your confidence grows.
   - *Healthy Cooking Methods*: Opt for cooking methods that preserve the nutritional value of your food, such as steaming, grilling, roasting, or sautéing. Avoid deep-frying or overcooking, which can reduce the nutrient content.

3. **Inspiration Sources**
   - *Online Resources*: Utilize food blogs, recipe websites, and social media platforms like Instagram and Pinterest for inspiration. Look for tags like #BrainHealthRecipes or #NeurogenesisDiet to find relevant ideas.
   - *Cookbooks*: Invest in cookbooks dedicated to brain health. Authors often provide valuable insights into the nutritional science behind the recipes along with practical tips for meal preparation.

- *Cooking Shows and Tutorials*: Watch cooking shows or online tutorials focused on healthy eating. Visual demonstrations can make it easier to understand new techniques and replicate them at home.

4. **Example Brain-Boosting Recipes**
    - *Salmon and Avocado Salad*: Combine grilled salmon, avocado slices, mixed greens, cherry tomatoes, and a sprinkle of walnuts. Dress with a lemon-tahini vinaigrette for a nutrient-packed meal.
    - *Quinoa and Veggie Stir-Fry*: Sauté garlic, onions, bell peppers, broccoli, and carrots in olive oil. Add cooked quinoa and a splash of tamari sauce. Top with sesame seeds and serve hot.
    - *Berry and Nut Smoothie*: Blend together a handful of spinach, mixed berries (blueberries, strawberries, raspberries), a tablespoon of flax seeds, and unsweetened almond milk. Enjoy as a refreshing breakfast or snack.

5. **Meal Planning and Preparation**
    - *Weekly Planning*: Set aside time each week to plan your meals. Create a shopping list based on the recipes you want to try. This ensures you have all the necessary ingredients on hand and

reduces the temptation to opt for less healthy options.
- ***Batch Cooking***: Prepare larger quantities of certain dishes and store leftovers in the fridge or freezer. This saves time and ensures you have healthy meals readily available on busy days.
- ***Portion Control***: Pay attention to portion sizes to avoid overeating. Use smaller plates and bowls if necessary to help manage portions visually.

By preparing healthy recipes that include a variety of brain-boosting ingredients, you can enjoy delicious meals while supporting your cognitive health. Experimentation and creativity in the kitchen can make the journey toward better brain health both fun and fulfilling.

Step 5: Monitor and Adjust Your Diet

Embarking on a new diet requires ongoing attention and flexibility to ensure it meets your needs effectively. Here's how you can monitor and adjust your dietary plan for optimal results:

1. **Track Your Progress**
    - ***Daily Journaling***: Keep a detailed log of your meals, snacks, and beverages. Note the time you eat, portion sizes, and any immediate feelings of satisfaction or hunger.

- *Weekly Reviews*: Set aside time each week to review your dietary logs. Look for patterns or trends that may indicate how well the diet is working for you.

2. **Assess Cognitive Function**
   - *Mental Clarity*: Pay attention to your ability to focus and concentrate throughout the day. Are you experiencing periods of brain fog or moments of heightened clarity?
   - *Memory Performance*: Notice any changes in your short-term and long-term memory. Are you recalling information more easily or struggling with forgetfulness?

3. **Evaluate Mood**
   - *Emotional Stability*: Monitor fluctuations in your mood. Are you feeling more even-tempered, or are there swings in your emotional state?
   - *Stress Levels*: Assess how your diet impacts your stress levels. Are you feeling more relaxed and resilient, or are you finding it harder to cope with daily pressures?

4. **Overall Well-being**
   - *Energy Levels*: Keep track of your energy throughout the day. Do you feel consistently energized, or are there times when you feel sluggish?

- *Physical Health*: Observe any physical changes such as weight loss or gain, changes in skin condition, or digestive issues.

5. **Make Necessary Adjustments**
   - *Nutritional Balance*: Ensure your diet provides a balanced intake of macronutrients (proteins, fats, carbohydrates) and micronutrients (vitamins, minerals). If you notice deficiencies, consider incorporating a wider variety of foods or supplements.
   - *Portion Sizes*: Adjust your portion sizes based on your energy requirements and satiety cues. Eating too little may leave you feeling deprived while overeating can cause discomfort and hinder progress.
   - *Hydration*: Keep hydrated by drinking sufficient water daily. Sometimes what we perceive as hunger is actually thirst.

6. **Seek Professional Advice**
   - *Dietitian Consultation*: Consult with a registered dietitian or nutritionist if you're unsure about adjusting your diet or if you experience persistent issues. They can provide personalized advice and help you fine-tune your meal plan.

By actively monitoring your diet and being ready to make adjustments, you can create a sustainable eating plan that supports both your cognitive function and overall well-being. Remember, the goal is to find a balance that works for you, ensuring long-term health and vitality.

Practical Tips for Shopping

Shopping for a healthy diet, especially one focused on brain health like the Neurogenesis Diet, requires some planning and strategy. Here are practical tips to help you shop effectively:

1. **Plan Ahead**
   - *Create a Meal Plan*: Outline your meals for the week before heading to the store. This will help you know exactly what ingredients you need and prevent impulsive purchases.
   - *Make a Shopping List*: Write down all the items you need based on your meal plan. Organize your list by sections of the store (e.g., produce, dairy, grains) to streamline your shopping trip.
2. **Shop Smart**
   - *Stick to the List*: Avoid buying items that aren't on your list. This helps you stay focused and within budget, reducing the temptation to purchase unhealthy foods.
   - *Shop on a Full Stomach*: Don't go grocery shopping when you're hungry; it can lead to impulse buys and unhealthy food choices.

3. **Focus on Whole Foods**
   - *Fresh Produce*: Prioritize fruits and vegetables, especially those known for their brain-boosting properties like berries, leafy greens, and avocados.
   - *Whole Grains*: Choose whole grains such as quinoa, brown rice, oats, and whole-wheat products over refined grains.
   - *Lean Proteins*: Incorporate sources of lean protein like fish (especially fatty fish like salmon), chicken, turkey, legumes, and tofu.
4. **Read Labels**
   - *Check Ingredients*: Look at the ingredient list of packaged foods. Opt for items with minimal ingredients and avoid those with added sugars, artificial additives, and unhealthy fats.
   - *Nutritional Information*: Pay attention to the nutritional labels to ensure you're meeting your dietary needs. Check for key nutrients like fiber, protein, vitamins, and minerals.
5. **Budget-Friendly Strategies**
   - *Seasonal Produce*: Buy fruits and vegetables that are in season; they are often fresher and more affordable.
   - *Bulk Buying*: Purchase non-perishable items like nuts, seeds, and whole grains in bulk to save money.

- ***Store Brands***: Consider store brand products, which are often cheaper than name brands and can be just as nutritious.

6. **Sustainability Practices**
   - ***Reusable Bags***: Bring your own reusable bags to reduce plastic waste.
   - ***Local Markets***: Shop at local farmers' markets where you can find fresh, locally grown produce. This supports local farmers and reduces the carbon footprint.

7. **Organizing Your Shopping Trip**
   - ***Start Perimeter***: Begin your shopping trip around the perimeter of the store where fresh foods like produce, dairy, and meats are usually located.
   - ***Limited Processed Foods***: Spend less time in the center aisles where processed and packaged foods are typically found.

8. **Additional Tips**
   - ***Frozen Options***: Stock up on frozen fruits and vegetables. They are convenient, have a long shelf life, and retain most of their nutrients.
   - ***Healthy Snacks***: Include healthy snack options like hummus, nut butter, yogurt, and fresh fruit to keep you satisfied between meals.

- ***Hydration Essentials***: Don't forget to buy items for hydration like herbal teas and sparkling water.

By following these practical shopping tips, you can efficiently stock your kitchen with healthy, brain-boosting ingredients that align with the Neurogenesis Diet. This will make it easier to prepare nutritious meals and maintain a healthy lifestyle.

Foods to Eat

When it comes to the Neurogenesis Diet, there are certain foods that are highly recommended due to their ability to support brain health and promote neurogenesis. These include:

1. **Fatty Fish**
- Rich in omega-3 fatty acids which support brain health
    - Salmon
    - Mackerel
    - Sardines
    - Trout

2. **Leafy Greens**
- High in vitamins, minerals, and antioxidants that protect neural function
    - Spinach
    - Kale
    - Swiss chard

- Collard greens

3. **Berries**
- Packed with antioxidants that help reduce inflammation and oxidative stress
    - Blueberries
    - Strawberries
    - Raspberries
    - Blackberries

4. **Nuts and Seeds**
- Good sources of healthy fats, vitamins, and antioxidants
    - Walnuts
    - Almonds
    - Flaxseeds
    - Chia seeds

5. **Whole Grains**
- Provide consistent energy and support overall brain function
    - Quinoa
    - Brown rice
    - Oats
    - Whole wheat

6. **Cruciferous Vegetables**
- Contains compounds that promote brain health and detoxification

- Broccoli
- Brussels sprouts
- Cauliflower
- Cabbage

7. **Legumes**
- Excellent sources of protein, fiber, and essential nutrients
    - Lentils
    - Chickpeas
    - Black beans
    - Kidney beans

8. **Healthy Fats**
- Support brain structure and function
    - Avocado
    - Olive oil
    - Coconut oil

9. **Herbs and Spices**
- Have anti-inflammatory and neuroprotective properties
    - Turmeric (curcumin)
    - Rosemary
    - Sage
    - Cinnamon

10. **Dark Chocolate**
- Opt for high-cocoa content (70% or higher)
- Contains flavonoids that enhance brain function

By incorporating these foods into your diet, you can support your brain health and overall well-being. Remember to also stay hydrated by drinking plenty of water and limiting your intake of processed and sugary foods.

Foods to Avoid

While certain foods can enhance brain function, others can have a negative impact. It's important to limit or avoid the following:

1. **Processed Foods**
- Often high in unhealthy fats, sugars, and additives that are detrimental to brain health
    - Fast food
    - Packaged snacks
    - Frozen meals
2. **Sugary Foods and Drinks**
- High sugar intake can lead to inflammation and impaired cognitive function
    - Sodas
    - Candy
    - Pastries
3. **Refined Carbohydrates**
- Cause spikes in blood sugar levels and offer little nutritional value
    - White bread
    - White rice

- Pasta made from refined flour

4. **Trans Fats**
- Linked to increased risk of brain diseases and poor cognitive function
    - Margarine
    - Fried foods
    - Certain baked goods

5. **Alcohol**
- Excessive consumption
- Can impair brain function and neurogenesis

6. **Artificial Sweeteners**
- Some studies suggest they may negatively impact brain health
    - Aspartame
    - Saccharin
    - Sucralose

7. **High-Sodium Foods**
- Excess sodium can lead to high blood pressure and negatively affect brain health
    - Processed meats
    - Canned soups
    - Snack chips

8. **Red Meat (in excess)**
- Limit intake of red meat like beef, pork, and lamb
- Choose lean cuts and moderate portions due to potential inflammatory effects

By focusing on these brain-boosting foods and avoiding those that can harm cognitive function, the Neurogenesis Diet aims to support and enhance brain health, promoting better memory, focus, and overall mental well-being.

Foods and Habits to Avoid

Now that you know which foods are best for this diet, it wouldn't benefit your efforts to improve if you were making lifestyle choices that impede the process. Here are some foods and habits you have to avoid if you're aiming for neurogenesis.

1. **Oxidized Vegetable Oils**

    We know in chapter 3 that oxidative stress hinders neurogenesis. In the making of seed and vegetable oils, high heat, pressure, and deodorizing processes make these oils edible. This process tends to strip away natural antioxidants that cause oxidative stress (Showdown, 2018).

    Coconut, canola, and sunflower-based cooking oil tend to have the lowest antioxidant content due to being stripped by the refinement process. Your better alternative would be to go for virgin olive oils in these cases.

2. **Foods high in refined sugar and fats**

   An excess in refined sugars and fats is known to cause cognitive decline and dementia (Knopman et al., 2001). These effects link to cardiovascular and cerebrovascular diseases (e.g., atherosclerosis). It's also known that these direct effects on the brain are proven.

   Although refined sugar and fats always make their way into our everyday dishes, moderation in intake is key to making sure we don't tax our body above what it can take. It is sound advice for all the things we consume.

3. **Alcohol**

   Intoxication through alcoholic beverages is known to inhibit neurogenesis in adults. (Geil et al., 2014). Studies have also shown that getting off any existing habit of drinking alcohol will increase the likelihood that new and healthy neurons are born.

4. **Opioid products**

   Opium originates from the white liquid of the Poppy plant. Although you won't find these in everyday meals, it would be best to avoid products that contain these. You also need to watch out for its tendency to have an addicting effect when consumed. Opioid products prevent the maturation and survival of newly born neurons (Zhang et al., 2016).

Week 1 – Meal and Stomach Prep

The transition from the usual diet to the Neurogenesis diet

Now, you likely have the basics down on what the diet is all about. You know what foods you can eat and what foods to avoid. You now know the basics to make it work. We'll now go through a 3-week guide to getting your body into the flow of the Neurogenesis diet.

Start with your gut

Switching diets isn't easy to do overnight. It is inadvisable to make extreme shifts in what you eat (Joshi & Mohan, 2018). For example, if you're going from a high-carb diet to a very low-carb all in one day, it can shock your system due to being unbalanced. Doing this also may not be sustainable in the long run.

Not a problem if your previous diet had the same nutritional profile or similar contents. But it would be best to ease into this new diet by eating your usual diet for the first two days of the week. Then, starting with the Neurogenesis-inducing meals on the third day onwards.

It would be helpful to do meal prep by pre-cooking the meats and fish rather than keeping them in the freezer. It will save time later on in the week and help you to stay on track. Here's a meal plan you can follow:

(Note: You can be creative, mix this up and be creative. Try out the recipes listed in Chapters 3 and 8 to keep your options fresh.)

Sunday

- Eat your usual diet

Monday

- Breakfast: Eat your usual diet
- Lunch: Salmon Soup. (See Chapter 8 for the recipe)
- Dinner: Garden greens salad with low-calorie dressing topped with blueberries

Tuesday

- Breakfast: Scrambled eggs on top of waffles and a side of avocado
- Lunch: Lightly chili-spiced rice topped with chickpeas
- Dinner: Pesto-sauce noodles topped with crushed walnuts.

Wednesday

- Breakfast: Oatmeal topped with mulberries and almond milk

- Lunch: Tortilla wraps filled with Greek yogurt, lettuce, and beans
- Dinner: Grilled beef burger with a side of steamed sweet potato

Thursday

- Breakfast: Raspberry Blueberry Smoothie (see Chapter 3 for recipe)
- Lunch: Cauliflower and chopped eggplant sautéed with garlic and onion
- Dinner: Braised salmon with a Green Tea Mango Blast (see Chapter 3 for the recipe)

Friday

- Breakfast: French toast topped with blueberries and Greek yogurt
- Lunch: Hot, hot, hot Salmon (see Chapter 3 for the recipe)
- Dinner: Avocado, Cucumber, and Tomato Salad (see Chapter 3 for the recipe)

Saturday

- Breakfast: Diced fruit salad with a side of hot green tea
- Lunch: Waffles topped with peanut butter and blueberry jam
- Dinner: Salmon Salad (see Chapter 3 for the recipe)

The good news about the Neurogenesis diet is that most foods you can eat can slot in quite nicely to whatever you were previously eating. If you're coming from your typical omnivorous diet, blueberries and salmon can be delicious options. If you're vegan, then curcumin, green tea, and avocados will do nicely. Your options for food aren't rigid. So, you have plenty of room for creativity.

Week 2 – Going Full Swing

Taking a Holistic Approach

Now that you've gone through a week of doing the neurogenesis diet, your mind and stomach more or less have a feel for what it's like to be eating to give your brain a boost to create more cells. Your next step is to incorporate some steps into your routine to complement the whole process of neurogenesis and general health. It's required to create an enriched environment in your brain to maximize survivability (Poulose et al., 2017). We'll go through the things you can add to your routine to do this:

Add Aerobic Exercise

No diet is complete without the stimulation of physical activity. The process of neurogenesis benefits the most when you're doing aerobic exercises (Nokia, 2016). The key is training your body to pump more oxygen to your brain.

If you're a beginner, start this week by going for a walk in the park. Doing this every day can already do wonders. In case you have a bicycle, whether stationary or for the road, you can hop on it and go for a stroll.

To get the most out of these aerobic activities, aim to increase the intensity every week. Start easy with up to 10-20 minutes at the start of the week. Then work toward adding a minute or more every week or so. The goal is to push yourself little by little every session, which also works for good cardiovascular health.

Doing cardio-type aerobic exercise also benefits the control of caloric balance for your body. That brings us to our following helpful routine.

Caloric Restriction

Adopting the neurogenesis diet is about eating right. It also means making sure you don't go overboard with your intake of calories (Poulose et al., 2017). When you map out your meal plan, you may also be careful not to eat too much or too little amounts of food. Using calorie-counting apps like MyFitnessPal can be helpful. You also avoid the risk of gaining or losing unnecessary weight when you mindfully track the calories you take in.

Cardio exercises do play an excellent role in caloric regulation. This week, start tracking your calories to be at least at maintenance level.

Sleep

Rest can be an overlooked part of being fit and healthy. People tend to want to do more or eat more rather than sleep to reach fitness goals. But it is one of the most vital parts of achieving optimal health, especially when going on a Neurogenesis diet.

Studies have shown that increased sleeping periods can increase cell genesis and survivability (Mueller et al., 2015). A lack of proper shut-eye can cause significant impairment in neurogenesis. Not getting enough sleep will also mess with your appetite levels and your energy for exercise.

An excellent rule of thumb is to aim for 8 hours of sleep for maximum recovery. Shoot for a good night's rest starting this week.

With these routine tweaks, you ensure up to 100% of newly created neurons survive into maturation and improve your lifestyle as a whole.

Since you've gone into full swing, you can now do the Full Swing Meal plan below. Don't be afraid to mix and shuffle it up to add some variety.

Sunday
- Breakfast: Sauteed beef with butternut squash and tomato soup

- Lunch: Chicken curry with chopped carrots, potatoes, and ginger
- Dinner: Blueberry Flax Smoothie (see Chapter 3 for recipe)

Monday

- Breakfast: Raspberry Blueberry Smoothie (see Chapter 3 for recipe)
- Lunch: Cauliflower and chopped eggplant sautéed with garlic and onion
- Dinner: Braised salmon with a Green Tea Mango Blast (see Chapter 3 for the recipe)

Tuesday

- Breakfast: Scrambled eggs on top of waffles and a side of avocado
- Lunch: Hot, hot, hot Salmon (see Chapter 3 for the recipe)
- Dinner: Avocado, Cucumber, and Tomato Salad (see Chapter 3 for the recipe)

Wednesday

- Breakfast: Diced fruit salad with a side of hot green tea
- Lunch: Waffles topped with peanut butter and blueberry jam
- Dinner: Salmon Salad (see Chapter 3 for the recipe)

Thursday

- Breakfast: Oatmeal topped with mulberries and almond milk
- Lunch: Salmon Soup. (See Chapter 8 for the recipe)
- Dinner: Grilled beef burger with a side of steamed sweet potato

Friday

- Breakfast: French toast topped with blueberries and Greek yogurt
- Lunch: Lightly chili-spiced rice topped with chickpeas
- Dinner: Pesto-sauce noodles topped with crushed walnuts.

Saturday

- Breakfast: Salmon with Avocados and Brussels sprouts (see Chapter 8 for the recipe)
- Lunch: Tortilla wraps filled with Greek yogurt, lettuce, and beans
- Dinner: Garden greens salad with low-calorie dressing topped with blueberries

Week 3 – Sustainability and Discipline

Once you've reached this week, you've likely gotten into the flow of the Neurogenesis diet. You've prepared and eaten the right foods, you've accompanied it with a good amount of exercise, and you've probably also fixed your sleep schedule. Your next goal is to make it last a lifetime.

If you've made it this far dedicating to this diet, it would be beneficial to stick with it for the long run. It's crucial to see the fruits of your discipline. But even if you're simply testing to see if this diet is the right one for you, you can still reap the benefits of feeding your brain with much-needed neurogenic foods.

At any rate, if you're determined to continue this diet further, in this chapter, we'll cover some key things you can do to achieve sustainability.

Set realistic goals (beyond the 3-week plan)

Since you already know what the Neurogenesis diet routine is like, you're more capable of making an educated approach to setting goals.

If your goal is to increase neurogenesis while also losing weight, you have to set a realistic number for how much weight you want to lose. Is it to lose half a pound every week? List that down. Is it to cut down on sugary snacks? Aim to only snack once every three days.

The point is to make it as realistic as possible. Don't put so high and out of reach. Manage your expectations from the get-go to ensure you stay on track and not give in early. It can help lower the chance of dropping out of a fitness program, especially if it's for weight loss (Dalle Grave et al., 2005).

Remove unhealthy foods from your house

You've gone to great lengths to improve what you eat. You don't want your efforts so easily disrupted by the mere sight of that yard-long Snickers bar stored in your fridge. It's possible to avoid unhealthy habits with the simple method of reducing or straight up throwing unhealthy foods out of your house.

It turns out that adults are affected by the mere sight of junk food that's within reach (Wansink et al., 2006). Think of the phrase "out of sight, out of mind," being able to discipline yourself to avoid the detrimental 6-pack of cold beer when it's not greeting you with every open of your refrigerator door. You'll be doing your new neurons and your liver a favor by shoving the temptation out the door.

Start by making an inventory of the food and drinks in your cupboard and fridge this week. List down the items that may trigger you to binge or return to old, unhealthy habits. Then proceed to throw them out, give them to a friend, or simply stop buying any more of them.

Track your progress

We already know we can't immediately see neurogenesis happening as we make the right choices. But the by-product of your other routine changes can be monitored by keeping a journal of your journey.

Studies have shown that short to long-term effects on weight loss can be enhanced with the use of health-tracking technology and coaches (Spring et al., 2013). Apps like MyFitnessPal or MyNetDiary are just some of the many free fitness tracking technologies you can use to help you maintain your integrity with your diet and the calories you're taking in. You can also be doing this with a friend who can coach you or do the Neurogenesis diet themselves. It adds a social aspect to your motivation that can push you to keep going.

For tracking actual brain improvement, you can look into narrative journaling. Just record in a notebook how you've been doing with your memory or problem-solving skills in everyday life. Maybe you can write down how much sharper you've been at the office during meetings. Perhaps you can record the scores you've been getting on quizzes you've taken at school.

If you're more into seeing how much your body's changed throughout the diet, you can take progress pictures. Some people get a boost in confidence seeing how much they've grown or cut down from comparing "before and after" images.

Recording and tracking will give you things you can look back on every once in a while. They can be a source of your motivation to sustain your healthy habits and help you carry them for decades down the line.

More Meal Ideas

If you're looking for more creative dishes to make for the Neurogenesis diet, here are a few more exciting recipes.

Salmon with Avocados and Brussels Sprouts

Ingredients:

- 4 salmon fillets
- 2 avocados, diced
- 1 cup Brussels sprouts, halved
- Salt and pepper to taste
- Olive oil for cooking

Instructions:

1. Preheat oven to 375°F (190°C).
2. Season salmon fillets with salt and pepper on both sides.
3. In a pan over medium-high heat, add olive oil and cook the salmon fillets for about 5 minutes per side or until golden brown.
4. Transfer the cooked salmon to a baking dish lined with parchment paper.
5. Spread diced avocados on top of the salmon fillets.
6. In the same pan, cook Brussels sprouts until slightly caramelized.
7. Add the Brussels sprouts on top of the avocados and season with salt and pepper.
8. Bake in the oven for 10-12 minutes or until salmon is cooked through and flaky.
9. Serve hot and enjoy!

Salmon Soup

Ingredients:

- 2 cups vegetable or chicken broth
- 1 cup water
- 1 pound salmon, cut into chunks
- 2 medium carrots, sliced
- 1 onion, diced
- Salt and pepper to taste

Instructions:

1. In a large pot, bring the broth and water to a boil.
2. Add the carrots and onions and let simmer for about 10 minutes.
3. Season with salt and pepper as desired.
4. Gently add the salmon chunks to the soup and cook for an additional 5 minutes or until the salmon is fully cooked.
5. Serve hot and enjoy!

Tortilla Wraps

Ingredients:

- 4 whole wheat tortilla wraps
- 1 cup Greek yogurt
- 1 head of lettuce, chopped
- 1 can black beans, drained and rinsed
- Salt and pepper to taste

Instructions:

1. In a bowl, mix together the Greek yogurt with salt and pepper.
2. Spread the mixture on each tortilla wrap.
3. Add a handful of chopped lettuce on top of the yogurt mixture.
4. Sprinkle black beans on top of the lettuce.
5. Roll up the tortillas tightly and cut in half for serving.
6. Serve cold or warm and enjoy!

French Toast

Ingredients:

- 8 slices of bread
- 4 eggs
- 1 cup milk
- 1 teaspoon vanilla extract
- Butter for cooking
- Fresh blueberries
- Greek yogurt

Instructions:

1. In a shallow dish, whisk together the eggs, milk, and vanilla extract.
2. Dip each slice of bread into the egg mixture, coating both sides.
3. Melt butter in a large pan over medium heat.
4. Cook the bread slices until golden brown on both sides.
5. Serve hot with a dollop of Greek yogurt and fresh blueberries on top.

Grilled Beef Burger

Ingredients:

- 1lb ground beef
- Salt and pepper to taste
- 4 burger buns
- Lettuce leaves
- Sliced tomatoes
- Sliced red onions
- Ketchup and mustard for toppings (optional)
- 2 medium-sized sweet potatoes, peeled and cut into cubes

Instructions:

1. Preheat a grill or grill pan on medium-high heat.
2. Season the ground beef with salt and pepper, then form into 4 equal-sized patties.
3. Grill the burgers for about 5 minutes on each side or until desired doneness.
4. While the burgers are cooking, steam the sweet potato cubes for about 10 minutes or until tender.
5. Assemble the burgers by placing a patty on each bun and topping them with lettuce leaves, tomatoes, and red onions.
6. Serve with ketchup and mustard if desired.
7. Drain any excess liquid from the steamed sweet potatoes and serve as a side dish to the grilled burger.

Pesto-Sauce Noodles

Ingredients:

- 1 package of spaghetti noodles
- 2 cups fresh basil leaves
- 1/4 cup pine nuts
- 3 cloves garlic, minced
- 1/2 cup grated parmesan cheese
- Salt and pepper to taste
- Olive oil for cooking
- Crushed walnuts for topping

Instructions:

1. Cook the spaghetti noodles according to the package instructions.
2. In a food processor, blend together the basil leaves, pine nuts, garlic, and parmesan cheese until smooth.
3. Slowly drizzle in olive oil while blending until the desired consistency is reached.
4. Season with salt and pepper to taste.
5. In a pan, heat up olive oil over medium heat and add the pesto sauce.
6. Add cooked spaghetti noodles to the pan and toss until fully coated in the pesto sauce.
7. Serve hot with crushed walnuts sprinkled on top for added crunch and flavor.

Waffles Topped with Peanut Butter and Blueberry Jam

Ingredients:

- 1 cup all-purpose flour
- 1 tablespoon sugar
- 2 teaspoons baking powder
- 1/4 teaspoon salt
- 1 egg, beaten
- 1 cup milk
- 2 tablespoons vegetable oil
- Peanut butter for topping
- Blueberry jam for topping

Instructions:

1. In a large mixing bowl, combine the flour, sugar, baking powder, and salt.
2. In a separate small bowl, beat the egg and mix in the milk and vegetable oil.
3. Pour the wet ingredients into the dry ingredients and mix until well combined.
4. Preheat a waffle iron and lightly coat with cooking spray.
5. Pour the batter into the waffle iron and cook according to the manufacturer's instructions until golden brown and crispy.

6. Top each waffle with a generous spread of peanut butter and blueberry jam before serving.
7. Optional: add some fresh blueberries on top for an extra burst of flavor.

Garden Greens Salad

Ingredients:

- Mixed greens (spinach, arugula, and/or romaine lettuce)
- 1/4 cup blueberries
- 1/4 cup chopped pecans
- Low-calorie salad dressing of choice (balsamic vinaigrette or lemon garlic recommended)

Instructions:

1. Rinse and dry the mixed greens.
2. In a large bowl, toss together the mixed greens with your desired amount of low-calorie dressing.
3. Top with fresh blueberries and chopped pecans.
4. Serve immediately as a side dish or add grilled chicken or tofu for a filling and healthy meal.

Tip: Toast the pecans in a pan over medium heat for a few minutes before adding to the salad for an extra crunch and depth of flavor.

Chicken Curry

Ingredients:

- 1 pound chicken breast, diced
- 2 tablespoons olive oil
- 2 cloves garlic, minced
- 1 small onion, chopped
- 2 carrots, peeled and chopped
- 2 potatoes, peeled and chopped
- 1 tablespoon grated ginger
- Salt and pepper to taste
- Curry powder to taste

Instructions:

1. In a large pan or pot, heat the olive oil over medium-high heat.
2. Add the diced chicken breast to the pan and cook until browned on all sides.
3. Remove the chicken from the pan and set aside.
4. In the same pan, add the minced garlic and chopped onion. Cook until translucent.
5. Add the chopped carrots and potatoes to the pan, stirring occasionally until they begin to soften.
6. Return the chicken to the pan and mix it with the vegetables.
7. Sprinkle curry powder over the mixture, using your desired amount for taste.

8. Add grated ginger, salt, and pepper to taste.
9. Continue cooking until all ingredients are fully cooked and flavors have combined.
10. Serve over rice or with naan bread for a complete meal that is full of flavor and nutrients.

Conclusion

Thank you for taking the time to journey through the Neurogenesis Diet Guide. By reaching the end of this guide, you've equipped yourself with powerful knowledge that can significantly impact your brain health and overall well-being.

By now, you've learned that neurogenesis, the process of generating new neurons in the brain, is not only possible but can be influenced by your dietary choices. This concept shifts the paradigm from simply maintaining brain health to actively enhancing it. The foods you consume have the power to foster a fertile environment for new neuron growth, which can improve cognitive functions such as memory, learning, and emotional regulation.

You've discovered the integral role of specific nutrients and foods in promoting neurogenesis. Omega-3 fatty acids, found in fish like salmon and flaxseeds, are essential for brain cell structure and function.

Antioxidant-rich fruits and vegetables, such as blueberries and spinach, protect your brain cells from oxidative stress and inflammation. Turmeric, with its active compound curcumin, not only adds flavor to your dishes but also spurs the creation of new neurons and enhances mood.

Furthermore, incorporating probiotics into your diet, whether through yogurt, kefir, or supplements, supports the gut-brain axis, demonstrating how interconnected our bodily systems truly are. Your gut health directly influences your brain health, showcasing the importance of a holistic approach to nutrition.

Adopting the Neurogenesis Diet involves more than just consuming specific foods; it's about making sustainable lifestyle changes. Regular physical activity, quality sleep, and stress management are all crucial components that complement your dietary efforts. Exercise increases blood flow to the brain, promoting the growth of new neurons.

Adequate sleep ensures that your brain has the restorative time it needs to consolidate memories and detoxify. Managing stress through mindfulness practices, such as meditation or yoga, creates an optimal mental environment for neurogenesis.

As you continue on your journey to better brain health, remember that consistency is key. The changes you've implemented should become long-term habits rather than short-lived trends. Start by integrating one or two new foods into your diet each week, gradually building up to a balanced and nutrient-dense regimen. Listen to your body, and adjust your diet to suit your individual needs.

The Neurogenesis Diet is not just about eating right; it's about nurturing your brain to achieve its full potential. It empowers you to take control of your cognitive health and actively contribute to your brain's longevity.

By embracing these principles, you pave the way for a sharper mind, improved emotional well-being, and a higher quality of life. In conclusion, we thank you for dedicating your time and effort to understanding the profound impact of your diet on neurogenesis. You are now equipped with the tools and knowledge to make informed decisions that will benefit your brain for years to come.

FAQs

What is neurogenesis, and why is it important?

Neurogenesis is the process of generating new neurons in the brain. This process is crucial for maintaining cognitive functions such as memory, learning, and emotional regulation. Promoting neurogenesis can help improve brain health, potentially delaying the onset of neurodegenerative diseases and enhancing overall mental well-being.

Which foods are most effective at promoting neurogenesis?

Foods rich in omega-3 fatty acids, antioxidants, flavonoids, and polyphenols are particularly effective at promoting neurogenesis. Examples include fatty fish like salmon, blueberries, dark chocolate, nuts, seeds, turmeric, green leafy vegetables, and fermented foods like yogurt and kefir.

How does exercise influence neurogenesis?

Regular physical activity increases blood flow to the brain, which helps deliver essential nutrients and oxygen that support the growth of new neurons. Exercise also stimulates the release of brain-derived neurotrophic factor (BDNF), a protein that encourages the development and maintenance of neurons.

Can stress negatively affect neurogenesis?

Yes, chronic stress can significantly hinder neurogenesis. High levels of stress hormones like cortisol can damage the hippocampus, a brain region critical for neurogenesis. Incorporating stress management techniques such as mindfulness, meditation, and yoga can help mitigate these negative effects.

How important is sleep for promoting neurogenesis?

Sleep is vital for neurogenesis. During sleep, your brain undergoes a variety of restorative processes, including the consolidation of memories and the clearance of toxins. Quality sleep ensures that your brain has the time it needs to repair and regenerate, facilitating the growth of new neurons.

Are there any supplements that can aid in neurogenesis?

Certain supplements may support neurogenesis, including omega-3 fatty acids (DHA), curcumin (found in turmeric), resveratrol (found in red grapes), and flavonoid-rich extracts like those from blueberries and green tea. However, it's important to consult with a healthcare provider before starting any new supplement regimen.

How soon can I see the benefits of following the Neurogenesis Diet?

The timeline for seeing benefits from the Neurogenesis Diet can vary depending on individual factors such as age, overall health, and consistency with the diet and lifestyle changes. Generally, improvements in cognitive function, mood, and overall brain health can be observed within a few weeks to months. Consistency is key; long-term adherence will yield the most significant benefits.

References and Helpful Links

Cortright, B. (n.d.). The neurogenesis diet and lifestyle: Upgrade your brain, upgrade your life. Digital Commons @ CIIS. https://digitalcommons.ciis.edu/facultypublications/3/

Grave, R. D., Calugi, S., Molinari, E., Petroni, M. L., Bondi, M., Compare, A., & Marchesini, G. (2005). Weight loss expectations in obese patients and Treatment attrition: an observational multicenter study. Obesity Research, 13(11), 1961–1969. https://doi.org/10.1038/oby.2005.241

Ding, M., Ma, H., Man, Y., & Lv, H. (2017). Protective effects of a green tea polyphenol, epigallocatechin-3-gallate, against sevoflurane-induced neuronal apoptosis involve regulation of CREB/BDNF/TrkB and PI3K/Akt/mTOR signalling pathways in neonatal mice. Canadian Journal of Physiology and Pharmacology, 95(12), 1396–1405. https://doi.org/10.1139/cjpp-2016-0333

Geil, C. R., Hayes, D. M., McClain, J. A., Liput, D. J., Marshall, S. A., Chen, K. Y., & Nixon, K. (2014). Alcohol and adult hippocampal neurogenesis: Promiscuous drug, wanton effects. Progress in Neuro-psychopharmacology & Biological Psychiatry, 54, 103–113. https://doi.org/10.1016/j.pnpbp.2014.05.003

Joshi, S., & Mohan, V. (2018). Pros & cons of some popular extreme weight-loss diets. Indian Journal of Medical Research, 148(5), 642. https://doi.org/10.4103/ijmr.ijmr_1793_18

Kim, G. H., Kim, J. E., Rhie, S. J., & Yoon, S. (2015). The role of oxidative stress in neurodegenerative diseases. Experimental Neurobiology/Experimental Neurobiology, 24(4), 325–340. https://doi.org/10.5607/en.2015.24.4.325

News-Medical. (2023, June 13). What is Neurogenesis? https://www.news-medical.net/health/What-is-Neurogenesis.aspx

Messick, G. (2023, August 1). The Neurogenesis Diet & Lifestyle Interview with author Brant Cortright, PhD. - Life Extension. https://www.lifeextension.com/magazine/2017/8/brant-cortright-phd-the-neurogenesis-diet-and-lifestyle

Mueller, A. D., Meerlo, P., McGinty, D., & Mistlberger, R. E. (2013). Sleep and Adult Neurogenesis: Implications for cognition and mood. In Current topics in behavioral neurosciences (pp. 151–181). https://doi.org/10.1007/7854_2013_251

Nokia, M. S., Lensu, S., Ahtiainen, J. P., Johansson, P. P., Koch, L. G., Britton, S. L., & Kainulainen, H. (2016). Physical exercise increases adult hippocampal neurogenesis in male rats provided it is aerobic and sustained. Journal of Physiology, 594(7), 1855–1873. https://doi.org/10.1113/jp271552

Poulose, S. M., Miller, M. G., Scott, T., & Shukitt-Hale, B. (2017). Nutritional factors affecting adult neurogenesis and cognitive function. Advances in Nutrition, 8(6), 804–811. https://doi.org/10.3945/an.117.016261

Knopman, D., Boland, L., Mosley, T., Howard, G., Liao, D., Szklo, M., McGovern, P., & Folsom, A. R. (2001). Cardiovascular risk factors and cognitive decline in middle-aged adults. Neurology, 56(1), 42–48. https://doi.org/10.1212/wnl.56.1.42

Sarker, M. R., & Franks, S. F. (2018). Efficacy of curcumin for age-associated cognitive decline: a narrative review of preclinical and clinical studies. GeroScience, 40(2), 73–95. https://doi.org/10.1007/s11357-018-0017-z

www.ingramcontent.com/pod-product-compliance
Lightning Source LLC
LaVergne TN
LVHW010410070526
838199LV00065B/5941